Renal diet cookbook

A Renal Diet Cookbook for Nourishing Kidney Health with Flavorful Precision

Dr. Juliet Newman

Copyright

This cookbook is designed to provide general information on renal diets and kidney-friendly recipes. It is not intended to be a substitute for professional medical advice, diagnosis, or treatment. Always seek the advice of your physician or other qualified health provider with any questions you may have regarding a medical condition. Never disregard professional medical advice or delay in seeking it because of something you have read in this cookbook.

Renal diet cookbook

A Renal Diet Cookbook for Nourishing Kidney Health with Flavorful Precision

Dr. Juliet Newman

Copyright

certain other noncommercial uses permitted by copyright law.

This cookbook is designed to provide general information on renal diets and kidney-friendly recipes. It is not intended to be a substitute for professional medical advice, diagnosis, or treatment. Always seek the advice of your physician or other qualified health provider with any questions you may have regarding a medical condition. Never disregard professional medical advice or delay in seeking it because of something you have read in this cookbook.

Introduction

In the quiet corridors of a bustling hospital, the story of the renal diet unfolds, weaving through the lives of individuals navigating the delicate terrain of kidney health. Meet Sarah, a resilient woman in her mid-fifties whose journey with chronic kidney disease (CKD) has become a testament to the transformative power of a meticulously crafted renal diet.

As the sun dipped below the horizon, casting a warm glow through the hospital room window, Sarah found herself grappling with the news of her CKD diagnosis. The somber tones of the doctor's words echoed in her mind, painting a vivid picture of a new reality filled with dietary restrictions and the need for mindful choices.

Enter the unsung hero of Sarah's narrative – the renal diet. What initially felt like an imposing set of rules soon unfolded as a lifeline, guiding her through the labyrinth of nutritional intricacies to safeguard her kidney function. The journey began with a gentle introduction to sodium management, an element that proved instrumental in maintaining blood pressure and fluid equilibrium.

The narrative of Sarah's dietary evolution expanded with the exploration of protein control – a delicate dance between nourishing her body with essential amino acids and relieving her kidneys of unnecessary strain. High-quality protein sources emerged as protagonists, offering sustenance without compromising the delicate balance her kidneys now required.

Phosphorus restriction, an aspect often overlooked in the broader dietary landscape, became a pivotal chapter. Sarah learned to decipher food labels with the precision of a detective, avoiding the hidden pitfalls of high-phosphorus foods that could impede her kidney's ability to function optimally.

As potassium regulation stepped into the limelight, Sarah faced the challenge of orchestrating a symphony of low-potassium alternatives, harmonizing them into a diet that catered not only to her taste buds but also to the intricate needs of her cardiac and renal health.

The narrative unfolded with fluid balance, a poetic exploration of hydration that went beyond mere sips of water. Sarah discovered the art of aligning her fluid intake with the ebb and flow of her body's needs, guarding against the perils of dehydration and fluid overload.

Calorie management, a chapter often overshadowed by the dietary intricacies, emerged as a beacon guiding Sarah toward a healthy weight. This, she discovered, was not merely about numbers on a scale but a fundamental aspect of supporting her kidneys on their arduous journey.

In the mosaic of Sarah's dietary journey, meal planning emerged as a canvas where each brushstroke contributed to a masterpiece of nourishment. Small, frequent meals became the rhythm of her days, a melody that resonated with the rhythm her kidneys needed to navigate the challenges ahead.

The narrative reached a crucial juncture with the careful avoidance of processed foods, known culprits laden with hidden phosphorus and potassium. Armed with the knowledge of discerning labels, Sarah embarked on a culinary adventure that embraced fresh, whole foods as the cornerstone of her renal diet.

Crucially, Sarah's story is not a solitary one but a collective narrative of resilience and adaptation. The renal diet, once perceived as a complex set of rules, revealed itself as a dynamic ally in her quest for kidney health. Through regular consultations with healthcare professionals, particularly the guiding hand of a registered dietitian, Sarah's dietary tale evolved, adapting to the twists and turns of her health journey.

In the symphony of Sarah's life, the renal diet emerged as a transformative overture, harmonizing nutrition, medical science, and personalized care. As the story unfolds further, the renal diet becomes more than a dietary paradigm – it transforms into a beacon of hope, guiding individuals like Sarah toward a future where the nuances of every meal contribute to the resilient tapestry of renal health.

Renal

The term "renal" refers to anything related to the kidneys. The kidneys play a crucial role in filtering waste and excess fluids from the blood to form urine. Conditions affecting the kidneys include chronic kidney disease (CKD), kidney stones, and various infections. A renal diet, as mentioned earlier, is designed to support kidney health by managing nutrient intake. Regular monitoring, medical attention, and lifestyle adjustments are essential for those with renal issues. If you have specific questions, feel free to ask.

Causes

There are various causes of renal (kidney) issues, including:

Chronic Kidney Disease (CKD): Often develops over time due to conditions like diabetes, hypertension, and glomerulonephritis.
Diabetes: Uncontrolled diabetes can damage the kidneys over time, leading to diabetic nephropathy.
Hypertension (High Blood Pressure): Prolonged high blood pressure can damage the small blood vessels in the kidneys, impacting their function.
Glomerulonephritis: Inflammation of the kidney's filtering units (glomeruli) can be caused by infections, immune system issues, or genetic disorders.
Kidney Stones: Formation of hard deposits in the kidneys, usually due to concentrated urine or imbalances in minerals.
Infections: Severe or recurring infections can lead to kidney damage.
Polycystic Kidney Disease (PKD): A genetic condition where fluid-filled cysts develop in the kidneys, affecting their structure and function.
Obstructive Disorders: Conditions like kidney tumors, enlarged prostate, or urinary tract obstructions can interfere with normal kidney function.
Autoimmune Diseases: Conditions such as lupus or certain types of vasculitis can affect the kidneys.
Trauma or Injury: Physical injury to the kidneys can impair their function.

Understanding the underlying cause is crucial for proper diagnosis and management of renal issues. Early detection and intervention can significantly impact outcomes. If you suspect kidney problems, consult a healthcare professional for proper evaluation.

Renal diet

A renal diet is tailored for individuals with kidney issues, focusing on managing sodium, potassium, and phosphorus intake. It often involves limiting high-potassium and high-phosphorus foods while ensuring adequate protein and fluid intake. Consultation with a healthcare professional or a registered dietitian is recommended for personalized guidance.

A renal diet is specifically designed to support kidney health, particularly in individuals with kidney conditions such as chronic kidney disease (CKD). Key aspects of a renal diet include:

Sodium Control: Limiting sodium helps manage blood pressure and fluid balance.

Protein Management: Controlling protein intake helps reduce the burden on the kidneys. High-quality protein sources are often recommended.

Phosphorus Restriction: Some renal patients need to limit phosphorus intake as impaired kidneys struggle to remove excess phosphorus.

Potassium Regulation: Monitoring and controlling potassium intake is essential, as imbalances can affect heart function.

Fluid Control: Adjusting fluid intake based on individual needs is crucial to prevent fluid retention.

Calorie Management: Maintaining a healthy weight through proper calorie intake is important.

It's crucial to personalize a renal diet based on individual health, stage of kidney disease, and specific nutritional needs. Consulting with a registered dietitian or healthcare professional is highly recommended for tailored guidance. Regular monitoring and adjustments to the diet are essential as kidney function changes over time.

Kidney friendly foods

Kidney-friendly foods are typically low in sodium, phosphorus, and potassium, and they support overall kidney health. Here are some examples:

Low-Potassium Fruits: Apples, berries, grapes, and pineapple are lower in potassium compared to bananas, oranges, and melons.

Vegetables: Choose low-potassium vegetables such as cabbage, cauliflower, bell peppers, and green beans. Limit high-potassium ones like potatoes and tomatoes.

Lean Proteins: Skinless poultry, fish, eggs, and small portions of lean meats are good protein sources with lower phosphorus content.

Dairy Alternatives: Opt for low-phosphorus milk substitutes like almond or rice milk instead of regular dairy.

Grains: Rice, pasta, and bread are generally lower in phosphorus. Choose whole grains in moderation.

Limit Processed Foods: Many processed foods are high in sodium, so opt for fresh, whole foods whenever possible.

Herbs and Spices: Use herbs and spices to add flavor without relying on salt.

Olive Oil: Use olive oil in moderation as a healthier alternative to other cooking oils.

Remember, individual dietary needs may vary based on specific health conditions and kidney function. Consultation with a healthcare professional or a registered dietitian is crucial for creating a personalized and effective kidney-friendly diet plan.

Meal plan

Creating a renal diet meal plan involves incorporating foods that are kidney-friendly and align with dietary restrictions. Here's a simple sample meal plan:

Breakfast:

Scrambled eggs with herbs (parsley, chives) - low in phosphorus

Toast made with white bread (instead of whole grain for lower phosphorus)

Apple slices (low in potassium)

Snack:

Greek yogurt (moderate protein, low phosphorus)

Berries (low in potassium)

Lunch:

Grilled chicken breast (lean protein, low phosphorus)

Quinoa or white rice (lower potassium option)

Steamed green beans (low potassium)

Snack:

Carrot sticks with hummus (moderate potassium, low
phosphorus)

Dinner:

Baked salmon (omega-3 fatty acids, moderate
phosphorus)

Mashed sweet potatoes (lower potassium than regular
potatoes)

Spinach salad with olive oil dressing (low potassium)

Dessert (in moderation):

Vanilla pudding made with low-phosphorus milk

Remember to adjust portion sizes based on individual nutritional needs and consult with a healthcare professional or a registered dietitian for personalized advice. Regular monitoring and adjustments to the meal plan may be necessary based on changes in kidney function.

Frequently asked questions

Here are some frequently asked questions (FAQs) regarding renal diets:

What is a renal diet?

A renal diet is a dietary plan designed to support kidney health, particularly for individuals with kidney conditions such as chronic kidney disease (CKD). It focuses on managing sodium, potassium, phosphorus, protein, fluid intake, and overall nutrition to lessen the burden on the kidneys.

Why is it important to follow a renal diet?

Following a renal diet helps manage symptoms, slow the progression of kidney disease, prevent complications such as electrolyte imbalances and fluid retention, and improve overall health and well-being.

What foods should I limit or avoid on a renal diet?

Foods high in sodium, potassium, phosphorus, and certain proteins should be limited or avoided. This includes processed foods, canned soups, high-potassium fruits and vegetables, high-phosphorus dairy, and red meats.

What are some kidney-friendly protein sources?

Lean meats (such as chicken and turkey), fish, eggs, tofu, and small portions of dairy are kidney-friendly protein sources. Plant-based proteins like beans and lentils can also be included in moderation.

How can I manage potassium intake on a renal diet?

Managing potassium intake involves choosing lower-potassium fruits and vegetables, leaching high-potassium vegetables, and moderating portion sizes. Boiling or soaking vegetables in water can help reduce their potassium content.

Are there specific cooking methods I should use on a renal diet?

Cooking methods such as grilling, baking, steaming, and boiling are recommended on a renal diet. These methods help retain nutrients while minimizing the need for added fats and sodium.

Can I still enjoy desserts on a renal diet?

Yes, but it's important to choose desserts that are lower in potassium, phosphorus, and sodium. Options include angel food cake, vanilla pudding made with low-phosphorus milk, and fruit sorbet.

How often should I consult with a dietitian when following a renal diet?

It's advisable to consult with a registered dietitian regularly to monitor your diet, adjust meal plans as needed, and address any concerns or challenges you may encounter while following a renal diet. Your healthcare team can help determine the frequency of these appointments based on your individual needs and health status.

Importance of nutrition on kidney health

Nutrition plays a crucial role in maintaining and promoting kidney health. The importance of nutrition in this context extends beyond mere sustenance, influencing the prevention of kidney-related issues and the management of existing conditions. Here are key aspects highlighting the significance of nutrition for kidney health:

Managing Chronic Kidney Disease (CKD):

For individuals with CKD, proper nutrition is instrumental in slowing the progression of the disease. A well-balanced diet helps alleviate the strain on compromised kidneys and minimizes complications associated with advanced stages of CKD.

Blood Pressure Regulation:

> Sodium, a component of salt, directly impacts blood pressure. By controlling sodium intake, individuals can manage blood pressure levels, reducing the risk of hypertension—a significant contributor to kidney damage.

Protein Balance:

> Protein is essential for the body, but excessive protein intake can strain the kidneys. Proper protein management ensures a balance between meeting nutritional needs and preventing the kidneys from working overly hard to eliminate waste products.

Phosphorus and Calcium Control:

> Imbalances in phosphorus and calcium can lead to mineral and bone disorders, common complications in kidney disease. Nutrition strategies that regulate phosphorus and calcium intake help maintain bone health and prevent complications.

Potassium Regulation:

Kidneys play a key role in balancing potassium levels in the body. Nutrition tailored to regulate potassium intake is crucial for preventing imbalances that can affect heart function and overall health.

Fluid Balance:

Adequate hydration is essential for kidney health. Maintaining the right fluid balance helps prevent dehydration or fluid overload, which can impact kidney function.

Managing Diabetes:

Diabetes is a leading cause of kidney disease. Nutrition, especially carbohydrate management, is vital for controlling blood sugar levels and reducing the risk of diabetic nephropathy.

Weight Management:

Maintaining a healthy weight is essential in preventing obesity-related kidney issues. Nutrition that supports weight management reduces the risk of developing kidney disease and supports overall well-being.

Reducing Oxidative Stress:

Antioxidant-rich foods help combat oxidative
stress, a factor implicated in kidney damage. A
diet high in fruits and vegetables contributes to
reducing oxidative stress and supporting kidney
health.

Preventing Kidney Stones:

Certain dietary factors, including inadequate fluid
intake and high consumption of oxalate-rich
foods, can contribute to kidney stone formation.
Proper nutrition can help prevent the
development of kidney stones.

In essence, a well-designed and individualized nutritional plan
is a cornerstone in the prevention, management, and overall
care of kidney health. Consulting with healthcare
professionals, particularly registered dietitians, ensures that
nutrition strategies are tailored to individual needs, considering
factors like age, overall health, and the specific stage of
kidney disease. Ultimately, prioritizing nutrition empowers
individuals to take an active role in preserving their kidney
health and fostering a better quality of life.

Tips for low sodium cooking

Cooking with low sodium is a key aspect of managing kidney health and overall well-being. Here are some tips for low sodium cooking:

Use Fresh Ingredients:

Opt for fresh fruits, vegetables, and meats instead of processed or pre-packaged options, which often contain high levels of sodium.

Read Labels:

When using packaged items, carefully read labels to identify sodium content. Choose products labeled as "low-sodium" or "no added salt."

Herbs and Spices:

Flavor your dishes with a variety of herbs and spices like basil, oregano, rosemary, and garlic to enhance taste without relying on salt.

Citrus Juices and Vinegar:

Use citrus juices (lemon, lime, orange) and vinegar to add acidity and flavor to your meals without increasing sodium levels.

Fresh or Dried Herbs:

Experiment with fresh or dried herbs like parsley, cilantro, thyme, or dill to add vibrant flavors to your dishes.

Homemade Seasoning Blends:

Create your own sodium-free seasoning blends by combining herbs, spices, and other flavor enhancers.

Limit Processed Foods:

Minimize the use of processed foods, as they often contain hidden sodium. Prepare meals from scratch using whole ingredients.

Rinse Canned Goods:

If using canned vegetables or beans, drain and rinse them thoroughly under cold water to remove excess sodium.

Cooking Methods:

Choose cooking methods like grilling, roasting, steaming, and baking to enhance natural flavors without relying on added salt.

Limit Salt in Recipes:

Gradually reduce the amount of salt you use in recipes. Your taste buds will adjust over time, and you may find that you need less salt than before.

Choose Low-Sodium Broths:

Use low-sodium or sodium-free broths and stocks when preparing soups, stews, and sauces.

Fresh Squeezed Citrus Zest:

Incorporate zest from citrus fruits to intensify flavor without adding sodium.

Explore Alternative Salts:

Experiment with alternative salts like potassium chloride, which can be a suitable substitute for those on low-sodium diets. However, consult with a healthcare professional before making significant changes.

Be Mindful of Condiments:

Many condiments, such as soy sauce and ketchup, can be high in sodium. Opt for low-sodium versions or use them sparingly.

Limit Use of High-Sodium Ingredients:

Foods like bacon, ham, and certain cheeses are high in sodium. Use them in moderation or explore low-sodium alternatives.

By incorporating these tips into your cooking routine, you can create flavorful, low-sodium meals that support kidney health and contribute to an overall heart-healthy lifestyle.

Protein rich kidney friendly recipes

Here are two protein-rich kidney-friendly recipes designed to support kidney health:

Grilled Lemon Herb Chicken

Ingredients:

- 4 boneless, skinless chicken breasts
- 2 tablespoons olive oil
- 2 tablespoons fresh lemon juice
- 2 teaspoons dried oregano
- 1 teaspoon dried thyme
- 1 teaspoon garlic powder

Salt and pepper to taste

Instructions:

Preheat the grill to medium-high heat.

In a bowl, mix together olive oil, lemon juice, oregano, thyme, garlic powder, salt, and pepper.

Brush the chicken breasts with the marinade, ensuring even coverage.

Grill the chicken for 6-8 minutes per side or until fully cooked.

Let the chicken rest for a few minutes before serving.

Quinoa and Vegetable Stir-Fry

Ingredients:

1 cup quinoa, rinsed

2 cups water

1 tablespoon vegetable oil

1 cup broccoli florets

1 bell pepper, thinly sliced

1 carrot, julienned

1 zucchini, sliced

2 cloves garlic, minced

1 teaspoon ginger, grated

2 tablespoons low-sodium soy sauce

1 tablespoon sesame oil

1 tablespoon rice vinegar

1 cup firm tofu, cubed (optional)

Instructions:

In a medium saucepan, bring water to a boil. Add quinoa, reduce heat to low, cover, and simmer for 15 minutes or until the quinoa is cooked and water is absorbed.

Heat vegetable oil in a large skillet over medium heat. Add broccoli, bell pepper, carrot, and zucchini. Sauté for 5-7 minutes until vegetables are tender-crisp.

Add minced garlic and grated ginger to the vegetables, cooking for an additional 1-2 minutes.

In a small bowl, whisk together soy sauce, sesame oil, and rice vinegar.

If using tofu, add it to the vegetable mixture and cook until lightly browned.

Add cooked quinoa to the skillet, pour the sauce over the mixture, and toss everything together until well combined.

Serve the quinoa and vegetable stir-fry hot, garnished with fresh herbs if desired.

These recipes provide protein from lean sources like chicken and tofu while incorporating kidney-friendly ingredients. Always consult with a healthcare professional or a registered dietitian to tailor recipes to your specific dietary needs and kidney health.

Phosphorus awareness

Phosphorus awareness is crucial, especially for individuals with kidney conditions, as it plays a significant role in maintaining bone health and other physiological functions. Here are key aspects of phosphorus awareness:

Function of Phosphorus:

Phosphorus is an essential mineral that plays a vital role in the formation and maintenance of bones and teeth. It is also involved in various cellular and metabolic processes.

Kidney Function and Phosphorus Regulation:

Healthy kidneys help regulate phosphorus levels in the blood by excreting excess phosphorus. However, impaired kidney function can lead to difficulty in eliminating phosphorus, resulting in elevated levels in the bloodstream.

Impact of High Phosphorus Levels:

Elevated phosphorus levels can contribute to mineral and bone disorders, leading to conditions such as bone pain, joint stiffness, and an increased risk of fractures. It can also contribute to cardiovascular complications in individuals with kidney disease.

Phosphorus in Foods:

Many foods contain phosphorus, and it's important to be aware of dietary sources. High-phosphorus foods include dairy products, nuts, seeds, whole grains, and certain meats.

Reading Food Labels:

Phosphorus may be present in various forms in processed and packaged foods. Reading food labels is essential to identify hidden sources of phosphorus, such as additives and preservatives.

Limiting High-Phosphorus Foods:

Individuals with kidney issues may need to limit high-phosphorus foods. This often involves reducing the intake of certain dairy products, organ meats, and processed foods.

Cooking Techniques to Reduce Phosphorus:

Certain cooking methods, like boiling or soaking high-phosphorus foods, can help reduce their phosphorus content. This is particularly relevant for beans and legumes.

Calcium-Phosphorus Balance:

Maintaining a proper balance between calcium and phosphorus in the diet is essential for bone health. Adequate calcium intake helps offset the impact of high phosphorus levels.

Phosphorus Binders:

In some cases, healthcare professionals may prescribe phosphorus binders. These medications help control phosphorus levels by binding to phosphorus in the digestive tract, preventing its absorption.

Consultation with Healthcare Professionals: Regular monitoring of phosphorus levels and consultation with healthcare professionals, including registered dietitians, are vital for developing a personalized dietary plan that addresses phosphorus awareness based on individual health and kidney function.

Awareness of dietary phosphorus is a key component of managing kidney health. Individuals with kidney conditions should work closely with healthcare professionals to tailor their dietary choices, ensuring a balance that supports overall well-being while mitigating the potential complications associated with elevated phosphorus levels.

Potassium regulations

Potassium regulation is essential for maintaining overall health, particularly for individuals with kidney conditions. Here are key aspects of potassium regulation:

Role of Potassium:

Potassium is a crucial mineral that plays a vital role in various physiological functions, including maintaining fluid balance, supporting proper muscle and nerve function, and regulating heartbeat.

Kidney Function and Potassium Balance:

Healthy kidneys help regulate potassium levels in the body by excreting excess potassium through urine. Impaired kidney function, as seen in conditions like chronic kidney disease (CKD), can lead to potassium imbalances.

Impact of High Potassium Levels (Hyperkalemia):

Elevated potassium levels in the blood, known as hyperkalemia, can have serious consequences, including irregular heartbeats or, in severe cases, cardiac arrest. Individuals with

kidney issues are at higher risk of hyperkalemia
due to reduced potassium excretion.

Potassium in Foods:

Many foods contain potassium, and awareness
of dietary sources is crucial. High-potassium
foods include bananas, oranges, potatoes,
tomatoes, and leafy green vegetables.

Reading Food Labels:

Reading food labels is essential to identify the
potassium content in processed and packaged
foods. Potassium-containing additives may be
present in certain products.

Limiting High-Potassium Foods:

Individuals with kidney conditions may need to
limit their intake of high-potassium foods. This
often involves reducing the consumption of
certain fruits, vegetables, and other potassium-
rich items.

Cooking Techniques to Reduce Potassium:

Cooking methods like boiling or leaching high-
potassium vegetables can help reduce their
potassium content. Soaking potatoes in water

before cooking is another method to lower their

potassium levels.

Balancing Potassium and Sodium Intake:

Maintaining a balance between potassium and

sodium intake is crucial for heart health.

Reducing sodium intake while ensuring an

adequate but controlled intake of potassium

contributes to this balance.

Individualized Dietary Plans:

Dietary plans for potassium regulation should be

individualized based on factors such as the

stage of kidney disease, overall health, and

specific nutritional needs. Consultation with a

healthcare professional, particularly a registered

dietitian, is essential.

Medication Management:

Some medications, such as certain blood

pressure medications, can affect potassium

levels. Individuals should communicate any

prescribed medications to their healthcare

providers to ensure a comprehensive approach

to potassium regulation.

Regular Monitoring:

Regular monitoring of potassium levels through blood tests is crucial for individuals with kidney issues. This allows healthcare professionals to make informed adjustments to dietary recommendations or medications.

Potassium regulation is a delicate balance that requires a thoughtful approach to dietary choices and lifestyle. Working closely with healthcare professionals, particularly registered dietitians, helps individuals with kidney conditions develop personalized strategies that support overall well-being while managing potassium levels effectively.

Calories management

Calorie management is a crucial aspect of a renal diet, especially for individuals with kidney conditions. Here are key considerations for calorie management in a renal diet:

Maintaining a Healthy Weight:

Calorie management is essential for maintaining a healthy weight. Excess body weight can contribute to complications in kidney health, so achieving and sustaining an appropriate weight is a primary goal.

Individualized Caloric Needs:

Caloric requirements vary among individuals based on factors such as age, gender, activity level, and overall health. Individualized assessment, often with the guidance of a registered dietitian, helps determine specific caloric needs.

Balanced Nutrition:

While managing calories, it's crucial to ensure that the diet remains balanced and provides essential nutrients. This includes adequate protein, vitamins, and minerals to support overall health.

Protein Intake Control:

Protein intake needs to be controlled, balancing the requirement for maintaining muscle mass while preventing excessive strain on the kidneys.

High-quality protein sources are prioritized, and portion control is emphasized.

Monitoring Portion Sizes:

Keeping an eye on portion sizes is key to calorie management. Smaller, more frequent meals may be recommended to distribute calorie intake evenly throughout the day.

Addressing Malnutrition Risk:

Individuals with kidney disease may be at risk of malnutrition, making it crucial to ensure that calorie intake meets nutritional needs. Calorie-dense, nutrient-rich foods can be incorporated to address this concern.

Adjustments Based on Health Status:

Caloric needs may change based on changes in kidney function, overall health status, or other factors. Regular monitoring and adjustments to the diet, if necessary, help maintain an optimal caloric balance.

Fluid Intake Considerations:

For some individuals with kidney conditions, managing fluid intake is part of the overall

dietary plan. Caloric beverages, if consumed,
contribute to overall caloric intake and should be
factored into the diet.

Collaboration with Healthcare Professionals:
Collaborating with healthcare professionals,
including registered dietitians, ensures a
comprehensive approach to calorie
management. Regular consultations allow for
adjustments to the dietary plan based on
individual health needs and changes in kidney
function.

Meal Planning for Balanced Calories:
Developing well-balanced meal plans that align
with individual caloric needs is crucial. Meal
planning helps individuals adhere to dietary
recommendations while enjoying a variety of
foods.

Physical Activity and Calorie Expenditure:
Considering physical activity levels is important
in calorie management. Adjustments to caloric
intake may be necessary based on individual
activity levels and goals.

Calorie management in a renal diet is not only about quantity but also about quality, ensuring that the calories consumed contribute to overall well-being while supporting kidney health. The collaborative effort between individuals, healthcare professionals, and registered dietitians helps tailor dietary plans to specific needs, fostering a holistic approach to managing kidney conditions.

Kidney friendly desserts recipes

Certainly! Here are two kidney-friendly dessert recipes that prioritize lower levels of phosphorus and potassium:

1. Baked Apple with Cinnamon and Walnuts

Ingredients:

- 2 apples (choose varieties with lower potassium content)
- 2 tablespoons chopped walnuts
- 1 teaspoon ground cinnamon
- 1 tablespoon honey (optional)

Instructions:

Preheat the oven to 375°F (190°C).

Wash and core the apples, leaving the bottom intact to create a well.

In a small bowl, mix chopped walnuts and ground cinnamon.

Fill each apple with the walnut-cinnamon mixture.

Place the apples in a baking dish and bake for approximately 25-30 minutes or until the apples are tender.

Drizzle honey over the baked apples if desired.

Serve warm and enjoy a comforting, kidney-friendly dessert.

2. **Berry and Greek Yogurt Parfait**

Ingredients:

1 cup mixed berries (strawberries, blueberries, raspberries)

1 cup low-fat or non-fat Greek yogurt

2 tablespoons chopped almonds (or seeds like
sunflower seeds)

1 teaspoon honey (optional)

Instructions:

Wash and prepare the mixed berries.

In a glass or bowl, layer Greek yogurt with mixed
berries.

Repeat the layers until you reach the top.

Top the parfait with chopped almonds or seeds.

Drizzle honey over the top if desired.

Refrigerate for a short time to chill or serve
immediately.

These desserts incorporate kidney-friendly ingredients and are
mindful of phosphorus and potassium content. As with any
dietary changes, it's essential to consult with a healthcare
professional or a registered dietitian to ensure that these
desserts align with individual dietary restrictions and health
needs.

Kidney friendly drinks

Choosing kidney-friendly drinks is important for individuals with kidney conditions, as certain beverages may impact fluid balance, electrolytes, and overall kidney function. Here are some guidelines for selecting kidney-friendly drinks:

Water:

Water is the best choice for maintaining proper hydration without adding extra calories, sodium, or other potentially harmful components. Adequate water intake supports kidney function and helps prevent dehydration.

Herbal Teas:

Unsweetened herbal teas are generally a safe choice. However, it's essential to avoid teas with ingredients that may be high in potassium, such as hibiscus or licorice root.

Coffee:

Coffee, when consumed in moderation, can be kidney-friendly. It's a low-calorie beverage that provides antioxidants. However, excessive

caffeine intake should be avoided, as it may
contribute to dehydration.

Fruit Juices (in moderation):

Some fruit juices can be included in moderation,
but it's crucial to choose those lower in
potassium. Additionally, diluting juices with water
can help reduce their potassium content.

Vegetable Juices:

Low-potassium vegetable juices can be a good
option. Be cautious with those containing high-
potassium vegetables like tomatoes or carrots.

Lemonade (with caution):

Lemonade made with a limited amount of lemon
juice and sweetened with a sugar substitute may
be suitable. However, excessive sugar intake
should be avoided, especially for individuals with
diabetes.

Low-Sodium Broth:

Low-sodium chicken or vegetable broth can be a
warm, savory option, especially in colder
weather. It helps contribute to fluid intake without
overloading on sodium.

Diluted Sports Drinks (occasionally):

For individuals engaging in physical activity, diluted sports drinks can help replenish electrolytes. However, they should be consumed occasionally and in moderation.

Limit Carbonated Beverages:

Carbonated beverages may contain phosphoric acid, which can contribute to phosphorus levels. It's advisable to limit intake and choose those without added phosphoric acid.

Avoid High-Potassium Beverages:

Be cautious with beverages high in potassium, such as certain fruit smoothies or coconut water, as they may contribute to elevated potassium levels.

Limit Alcoholic Beverages:

Alcohol can affect kidney function and interact with medications. It's crucial to limit alcohol intake and consult with healthcare professionals about its compatibility with individual health conditions.

Always consult with a healthcare professional or a registered dietitian to determine the most suitable beverages for individual dietary needs and kidney health. Regular monitoring of kidney function, fluid balance, and electrolyte levels helps ensure the chosen drinks align with overall health goals.

Summary

A renal diet, also known as a kidney-friendly diet, is specifically designed to manage the nutritional needs of individuals with kidney conditions, especially chronic kidney disease (CKD). Here's an overview covering various aspects of a renal diet:

Sodium Management:

Sodium intake is often restricted to manage blood pressure and fluid balance. This involves minimizing processed and high-sodium foods.

Protein Control:

Controlling protein intake is crucial to reduce the load on the kidneys. High-quality protein sources with essential amino acids are emphasized.

Phosphorus Restriction:

Phosphorus levels are monitored, as impaired kidneys struggle to excrete excess phosphorus. Foods high in phosphorus, such as dairy and certain meats, may be limited.

Potassium Regulation:

Managing potassium is essential to prevent imbalances that can affect heart function. High-potassium foods, like bananas and oranges, might be restricted, while lower-potassium alternatives are encouraged.

Fluid Balance:

Maintaining an appropriate fluid balance is crucial. The recommended fluid intake varies

depending on factors like individual health and
stage of kidney disease.

Calorie Management:

Adjusting caloric intake is important to maintain a
healthy weight. A dietitian can help determine
appropriate calorie levels based on individual
needs.

Meal Planning:

Meal plans often focus on small, frequent meals
to avoid overloading the kidneys. Balancing
carbohydrates, proteins, and fats is essential for
overall nutrition.

Limiting Phosphorus and Potassium in Processed
Foods:

Processed foods, often high in phosphorus and
potassium additives, are limited. Reading food
labels becomes crucial to identify hidden
sources.

Cooking Methods:

Cooking methods like baking, grilling, steaming,
and boiling are preferred to minimize added fats
and sodium.

Individualization:

A renal diet is highly individualized. Factors like the stage of kidney disease, overall health, and specific nutritional needs influence dietary recommendations.

Consultation with Healthcare Professionals:

Regular consultation with healthcare professionals, particularly registered dietitians, is crucial. They can provide personalized advice, monitor nutritional status, and adjust dietary plans as needed.

Adherence to a renal diet, along with medical management, can help slow the progression of kidney disease, manage symptoms, and enhance overall well-being for individuals with renal issues.

Conclusion

In conclusion, adopting and adhering to a renal diet is a pivotal
component in the comprehensive management of kidney
health, particularly in the context of chronic kidney disease
(CKD) and related conditions. The intricacies of this dietary
approach revolve around meticulous control over sodium,
phosphorus, potassium, protein, and fluid intake. Each
element is carefully tailored to alleviate the strain on
compromised kidneys, slow the progression of the disease,
and enhance overall well-being.

Sodium management serves as a linchpin, not only in blood
pressure regulation but also in preserving fluid balance. By
curbing sodium intake, individuals with kidney issues can

mitigate the risk of edema and hypertension, common complications associated with impaired renal function.

Protein control assumes a nuanced role, striking a delicate balance between providing essential amino acids and reducing the burden on the kidneys. Opting for high-quality protein sources, coupled with moderation, becomes paramount to achieving this equilibrium.

Phosphorus restriction is imperative, recognizing the kidneys' challenge in effectively excreting excess phosphorus. This often involves meticulous scrutiny of food labels and a conscious effort to limit high-phosphorus foods, such as certain dairy products and meats.

Potassium regulation, another cornerstone of the renal diet, is vital in averting potentially serious imbalances that could compromise cardiac function. Through the selective inclusion of low-potassium alternatives and judicious portion control, individuals can manage this essential mineral effectively.

Fluid balance, often overlooked, plays a crucial role in kidney health. Striking the right balance in fluid intake, tailored to individual needs and disease stage, is essential for preventing complications associated with fluid overload or dehydration.

Calorie management underscores the importance of maintaining a healthy weight, acknowledging that excess body weight can exacerbate kidney-related issues. This aspect of the renal diet is a holistic approach to overall health and well-being.

Meal planning in a renal diet emphasizes small, frequent meals to avoid overwhelming the kidneys. Balancing macronutrients—carbohydrates, proteins, and fats—ensures comprehensive nutrition while aligning with the dietary restrictions necessary for kidney health.

The meticulous avoidance of processed foods, known for their high phosphorus and potassium content, adds another layer of complexity to the renal diet. This necessitates a vigilant approach to reading food labels and making informed choices to sidestep hidden sources of these minerals.

Crucially, the renal diet is not a one-size-fits-all paradigm. Instead, it's a highly individualized approach that takes into account the unique circumstances of each individual—

considering factors such as the stage of kidney disease, comorbidities, and overall nutritional requirements.

Regular consultation with healthcare professionals, particularly registered dietitians, becomes a cornerstone in the successful implementation of a renal diet. Their expertise ensures that dietary plans are not only effective but also adaptable to changes in kidney function, overall health, and individual needs.

In embracing the principles of a renal diet, individuals can empower themselves to play an active role in managing their kidney health. Through this dietary strategy, they gain a tool for slowing the progression of kidney disease, alleviating symptoms, and fostering an improved quality of life. As a comprehensive and holistic approach, the renal diet stands as a testament to the intersection of nutrition, medical science, and patient-centric care in the realm of renal health. It's